Low Cholesterol Diet
How to Lower Your Cholesterol Naturally to Prevent and Reverse Heart Disease

Table of Contents

Introduction

Dear reader,

I want to thank you and congratulate you for buying the book, "Low Cholesterol Diet - How To Lower Your Cholesterol Naturally to Prevent and Reverse Heart Disease".

When writing this book, our main target was to help you to reduce your cholesterol naturally without "torturing" you and your body with the classic weight losing diet. Moreover, cholesterol is not about limiting your meal; it's about replacement of fats with healthy food products and changing your lifestyle.

Reducing cholesterol naturally requires a complex approach to what you eat and do in your everyday life. The book will help and guide you through this process and will provide you with useful tips and diet recipes that will help you to decrease the level of cholesterol in your blood and simply become a healthy person. And as the ancient Roman poet Juvenal once said, **Mens sana in corpora sano** or *"A sound mind in a sound body."*

Hope this book will be helpful and valuable in shaping your future healthy life.

Thanks again for buying this book, I hope you enjoy it!

Chapter 1 - A Few Facts about Cholesterol

Before speaking about the advantages and risks of cholesterol, first all of we should realize that cholesterol is the integral part of our bodies. Cholesterol is a hydrocarbon organic molecule biosynthesized by cells of all types of animals, including humans. It's the vital structural part of membranes which ensures its structural integrity and fluidity. There's HDL cholesterol ("good") and LDL cholesterol ("bad") and they perform different functions.

High-density lipoproteins (HDL) are small molecules that pick up excess cholesterol in the blood and take back to the liver. Low-density lipoproteins (LDL) carry cholesterol throughout the body, transporting it to different organs and tissues. But if you have too much cholesterol, then is it is necessary for this process that the excess keeps circulating in your blood and the LDL deposits the cholesterol into the arteries. This can lead to blockages and cause heart attacks. That's why LDL is often referred to as the "bad" cholesterol.

But the same way as in nature, the human body also requires a balanced proportion of cholesterol in your blood. Any deviation from its limits may and will lead to health related risks. Taking into account the fact that the most of today's world population suffers from high cholesterol levels because of consuming unhealthy junk food, this book will focus on reduction of cholesterol in your organism and bringing back its glory.

Reading medical books you will find out that the level of cholesterol often increases with age thus presenting certain risks for cardiologic or simply heart diseases. You'll need to undergo periodical examinations and sometimes your physician will prescribe you certain medicine to keep the cholesterol level within acceptable limits.

And here the good news is that there is safer and simpler way for natural reduction of cholesterol!

Chapter 2 - A Few Tips on How to Reduce Cholesterol Naturally

As you have already realized, this book and tips, as well as recipes below are not just simple dietary plans you need to follow. First of all, you need to understand that you should adopt healthy lifestyle, balanced eating and exercises which is the vital part of this process. You should consider replacing high cholesterol food with low cholesterol as well as cholesterol-lowering food products.

Below, you can find useful and valuable tips for reducing your cholesterol:

1. **Decrease meat intake.** Make it minor part of your meal. Avoid meat fats and skins which contain high level of cholesterol! Consider replacing meat product with fish or meatless pasta.

2. **Try low fat varieties of your favorite dairy products!** If you like dairy products like milk, choose one that contains lower level of fat and cream.

3. **Re-think about snacks!** Again, lower fat snack (dried fruits, vegetables, carrots etc) are more preferable and healthier than those you buy in store like potato chips, candy bars, etc.

4. **Don't use saturated fat in your meal!** Saturated fat like butter and margarine can be well replaced by liquid oils.

5. **Use healthy oils.** Olive oil and rapeseed oil contain mainly monounsaturated fats, so they are always a good choice for healthy cooking. They help to make the artery walls stronger and decrease the risk to be damaged by cholesterol. Nutritional experts confirmed that daily consumption of 2 tablespoons of olive oil would decrease total cholesterol by eight per cent in six weeks. Palm and coconut oilscontain

saturated fat unlike other vegetables so avoid using these two oils. Generally, studies suggest that virgin olive oil is best.

6. ***Increase intake of foods rich in soluble fiber!*** Grain products (barley, oats), legumes (beans, peas) are rich in *soluble fiber,* which helps your body eliminate cholesterol. Try to start your day with a bowl of old-fashioned oats. Use barley and black beans in your soups.

7. ***Eat more fruits and vegetables!*** Fruits and vegetables are good sources of heart-healthy antioxidants and they are also rich in cholesterol-lowering dietary fiber.

8. ***Eat more fish!*** As you may know, fish contains acids namely Omega-3s and Omega-6s, which your body doesn't generate. Those acids will help to reduce your blood pressure, as well as the risk of developing blood clots, thus improving the level of your cholesterol. Make sure to use baked or grilled fish to avoid adding unhealthy fats.

9. ***Use nuts!*** Nuts are a good source of proteins, fiber, heart healthy unsaturated fats, vitamin E. Walnuts, almonds and other nuts can reduce blood cholesterol. But be careful with overuse of nuts, as they may cause weight gain due to their caloric content. To avoid weight gain, substitute foods rich in saturated fat with nuts. For example, instead of using meat, cheese, or mayo in your salad, add a handful of walnuts or almonds.

10. ***Reduce intake of cholesterol in your meal!*** If you want cholesterol-lowering foods work effectively, it makes sense to limit foods that can raise your cholesterol level. Try to use not more than 200 mg of cholesterol daily. Limit your intake of eggs, meat, poultry and other fat-rich products.

11. ***Avoid trans fats!*** Trans fats are a real danger for your health. They raise your "bad" (LDL) cholesterol level and decrease the amount of "good" (HDL) cholesterol. So avoid or use as much as possible smaller portions of foods that contain trans fats.

1. It's time to change your habits

    1. ***Reduce salt intake!*** Salt provokes high blood pressure and creates risks for heart diseases. So think about cutting down salt intake.

    2. ***Limit drinking alcohol!*** Reasonable use of alcohol, especially red wine, can be beneficial in decreasing risks related to heart disease but overuse of alcohol can have the opposite effect. It's recommended to have one drink per day for women and one or two drinks for men.

    3. ***Quit smoking!*** Smoking lowers good cholesterol (HDL) and raises bad cholesterol (LDL). It also damages your arteries, increases the risk of heart diseases, such as high blood pressure and diabetes. Studies have shown that cholesterol profiles improve after a person quits smoking.

    4. ***Read carefully the list of ingredients on the food before buying it!*** Foods made of such ingredients as palm or coconut oil, butter, margarine, lard, cocoa butter are main "companions" of cholesterol. Avoid also fast food and food containing hydrogenated or partially hydrogenated fat or oil.

    5. ***And eventually get active!*** An active lifestyle is one of the most important guarantees for lowering you cholesterol level. Start walking, cycling, running and dancing, as well as consider aerobic exercises which will not only keep you in a good and beautiful shape but also improve your heart conditions.

To make your life easier, the section below offers you several health recipes designed for your breakfast, lunch and dinner and which will guide you through the process of reducing the cholesterol in your blood. Recipes are easy to cook and contain accessible ingredients which you can find everywhere. All recipes are based on tips and products mentioned above.

Chapter 3 - Breakfast Recipes

1. Muffins

Prep time: 5 minutes

Cook time: 20 minutes

Nutritional information per serving: Calories 109.5; Fat 2.9 g; Cholesterol 0.5 mg.

Serves 12.

Ingredients

- 2 1/4 cup oat bran cereal (finely ground)
- 1/4 cup nuts, chopped (walnuts/pecans)
- 1/4 cup dates, chopped (or raisins)
- 1 tsp baking powder
- 1/4 cup packed brown sugar or ¼ cup honey 1
- 1/4 cup skim milk
- 2 egg whites or 2 egg substitute.
- 2 tbs. vegetable oil (or canola oil-no olive oil)

Directions

- Place the nuts, dates, oat bran cereal and baking powder in a large bowl. Stir in the brown sugar or ¼ cup honey.
- In a medium bowl, gently whisk the egg whites, milk and oil and combine with the oat bran mixture. Mix until well blended.
- Gently coat the muffin tin with cooking spray or line with paper cups. Then spoon the batter into muffin cups and bake for 15-20 minutes or until the toothpick inserted in the batter of the muffin comes out clean.

- You may store muffins in a plastic bag in the refrigerator or freeze for longer storage.

2. Oatmeal-Rhubarb Porridge

Prep time: 10 minutes

Cook time: 10 minutes

Nutritional information per serving: Calories 336; Fat 8 g; Cholesterol 4 mg.

Serves 2.

Ingredients:

- 1/2 cup orange juice
- Pinch of salt
- 1 1/2 cups nonfat milk or nondairy milk (soymilk or almond milk)
- 1 cup old-fashioned rolled oats
- 1 cup 1/2-inch pieces rhubarb, fresh or frozen
- 1/2 tsp ground cinnamon
- 2-3 tbs brown sugar or pure maple syrup
- 2 tbs pecans or other nuts (toasted, chopped)

Directions:

1. Add oats, milk, rhubarb, juice, and cinnamon in a medium saucepan, season with a pinch of salt and bring to a boil over medium-high heat.
2. Then reduce heat, put the lid on and allow it to simmer, stirring frequently, until the oats and rhubarb are soft, about 5 minutes.

3. Remove the pan from the heat and let stand for at least 5 minutes, covered. Stir in the sugar or syrup to taste. Place the porridge in a serving bowl, sprinkle with nuts and enjoy.

3. Quinoa with Peaches and Creamy Yogurt

Prep time: 5 minutes

Cook time: 20 minutes

Nutritional information per serving: Calories 219; Fat 3 g; Cholesterol 0 mg.

Serves 4

Ingredients:

- 1 cup quinoa
- 2 cups water
- 1 tsp ground cinnamon
- 1 tsp ground nutmeg
- 1 large fresh peach (pitted, chopped)
- 1/2 cup fat-free Greek yogurt
- 2 tbs honey (or to taste)
- 1 pinch ground nutmeg

Directions:

1. Rinse quinoa in the cold water and drain.

2. Add quinoa to 2 cups of boiling water and let cook over low heat until it has softened, about 15-20 minutes. Pour off the excess water, if left and stir in the nutmeg and cinnamon.

3. In a small bowl, combine the yogurt and peach and mix well. Place the cooked quinoa in serving bowls, top with 2 tbs of peach yogurt, drizzle with about 1 tsp honey, season with ground nutmeg and enjoy.

4. Breakfast Barley with Banana and Sunflower Seeds

Prep Time: 5 minutes
Cook Time:15 minutes
Nutritional information per serving: Calories 410,Fat 6 g,Cholesterol 0 mg.

Serves 1

Ingredients:

- 2/3 cup water
- 1/3 cup uncooked quick-cooking pearl barley
- 1 banana (sliced)
- 1 tsp honey
- 1 tbs unsalted sunflower seeds

Directions:

1. Place barley in a small microwave-safe bowl, add 2/3 cup of water and microwave at high for 6 minutes.

2. Give a stir and let stand for about 5 minutes.

3. Place the barley in a serving bowl, top with banana slices and honey, sprinkle with sunflower seeds and enjoy.

5. Omelet Cups

Prep Time: 35 minutes

Cook Time: 25 minutes

Nutritional information per serving: Calories 28, Fat 0.13g, Cholesterol 0 mg.

Serves 6

Ingredients:

- 1/2 cup red onion, (chopped)
- 1/2 cup bell peppers (chopped)
- 1 cup egg white
- 1 dash black pepper
- 1/2 cup mushrooms (sliced)

Directions:

1. Preheat oven to 350 °F (175 °C)
2. Line the muffin tin with paper liners.
3. In a large bowl beat egg whites until smooth. Stir in the mushrooms, onions and bell peppers and mix well to combine.
4. Fill a muffin tin about 3/4 way full and bake in the oven about 25 minutes or until egg is cooked.

6. Breakfast Bulgur Porridge

Prep time: 5 minutes

Cook time: 15 minutes

Nutritional information per serving: Calories 340; Fat 6.7g; Cholesterol 12mg.

Serves 4.

Ingredients:

- 4 cups low-fat (1%) milk
- 1 cup bulgur
- 1/3 cup dried cherries
- 1/4 teaspoon salt
- 1/3 cup dried apricots, coarsely chopped
- 1/3 cup sliced almonds

Directions:

1. Add the bulgur, milk, dried cherries to a medium saucepan and set over medium- high heat. Once boiling, slow down the heat and let cook, stirring often, until the bulgur has softened, 10-15 minutes.

2. Season with salt, give a stir and remove from the heat.

3. Ladle the porridge into serving bowl, garnish with almonds and dried apricots and enjoy.

7. Apple-Cinnamon Granola

Prep Time: 10 minutes
Cook Time:1 hr 40 minutes
Nutritional information per serving: Calories 196,Fat 5 g,Cholesterol 5 mg.

Serves 6

Ingredients:

- 3 cups regular oats
- 1 cup whole-grain toasted oat cereal
- 1/3 cup oat bran
- 1/3 cup finely chopped walnuts
- 2 tsp ground cinnamon
- 1/4 tsp ground cardamom
- 2 tbsp butter
- 1/3 cup applesauce
- 1/4 cup honey
- 2 tbsp brown sugar
- Cooking spray
- 1 cup dried apple, chopped

Directions:

1. Preheat oven to 250°F (120 °C).
2. In a large bowl, place together the oats, oat bran, toasted oat cereal, walnuts, cardamom and cinnamon. Mix well to combine.
3. Add 2 tablespoons butter to a medium pot and heat over medium heat.

4. Add honey, brown sugar 1/3 cup applesauce to a skillet and set over moderate heat. Once it begins to bubble, give a stir and pour the mixture over mixed oats.

5. Coat a rimmed baking sheet with cooking spray.

6. Transfer the mixture to the prepared baking sheet and bake in the oven for about 1 1/2 hours, stirring 2-3 times, approximately every 30 minutes.

7. Withdraw from the oven and let cool completely.

8. Add the chopped apple, mix to combine.

9. Place the granola into serving bowls and enjoy.

8. Banana Breakfast Smoothie

Prep time: 5 minutes

Nutritional information per serving: Calories 212; Fat 3.6; Cholesterol 9mg.

Serves 1.

Ingredients:

- 1/2 cup 1% low-fat milk
- 1 tbs honey
- 1/8 tsp ground nutmeg
- 1 frozen ripe large banana, sliced
- 1 cup plain 2% reduced-fat Greek yogurt

Directions:

- In a blender, add the milk, nutmeg, honey and banana, then pulse 1-2 minutes until fluffy and smooth.
- Stir in the yogurt, pulse for a few seconds. Pour the mixture into a serving glass and enjoy.

9. Healthy Nutty Granola

Prep time: 5 minutes

Cook time: 30 minutes

Nutritional information per serving: Calories 279; Fat 11 g; Cholesterol 0 mg.

Serves 9.

Ingredients

- 1/3 second canola cooking spray
- 3 cups dry old-fashioned oats
- 1/2 cup shelled walnuts
- 1/2 cup raisins
- 1/2 cup maple syrup
- 1/4 tsp cinnamon
- 1/4 tsp salt
- 1/2 cup, slivered almonds
- 1/2 cup pecans (halves)

Directions:

1. Preheat oven to 350 °F (175 °C). Gently oil a baking sheet with cooking spray.
2. In a large bowl, place together the old-fashioned oats, raisins, walnuts, almonds, pecans, cinnamon, salt and maple syrup.
3. Mix well to combine.
4. Place the mixture in the baking sheet and bake in the oven for 25-30 minutes, stirring 2-3 times. Remove from the oven and let cool completely.

5. Let stand in the refrigerator for at least 2 hours before serving.

10. Quinoa risotto with arugula and Parmesan

Prep time: 5 minutes

Cook time: 20 minutes

Nutritional information per serving: Calories 147; Fat 3 g; Cholesterol 3 mg.

Serves 6

Ingredients

- 1 tablespoon olive oil
- 1/2 yellow onion, chopped
- 1 garlic clove, minced
- 1 cup quinoa, well rinsed
- 2 1/4 cups vegetable broth
- 2 cups arugula, chopped, stemmed (rocket)
- 1 small carrot, peeled, finely shredded
- ½ cup thinly sliced fresh shiitake mushrooms
- ¼ cup Parmesan cheese, grated
- ½ tsp salt
- ¼ tsp freshly ground black pepper

Directions

1. Add the olive oil to a large griddle and set over medium heat. Stir in the onion and cook for about 5 minutes, until tender.

2. Stir in the garlic, cook sauté for a minute and then add the quinoa. Sauté for 1-2 minutes, stirring frequently.

3. Pour in the broth and bring the mixture to a boil. Slow down the heat and let simmer until the quinoa has just softened, about 10 minutes.

4. Add the onion and sauté until soft and translucent, about 4 minutes. Add the garlic and quinoa and cook for about 1 minute, stirring occasionally. Don't let the garlic brown.

5. Add the shredded carrot, arugula and mushrooms and cook for about 2-3 minutes. Once the quinoa grains become translucent, add the cheese, season with salt and pepper and remove from the heat.

6. Place the quinoa into a serving bowl and serve hot.

11. Buckwheat pancakes

Prep time: 5 minutes

Cook time: 20 minutes

Nutritional information per serving: Calories 143; Fat 3 g; Cholesterol 0 mg.

Serves 6

Ingredients

- 2 egg whites
- 1 tablespoon canola oil
- 1/2 cup fat-free milk
- 1/2 cup all-purpose (plain) flour
- 1/2 cup buckwheat flour
- 1 tablespoon baking powder
- 1 tablespoon sugar
- 1/2 cup sparkling water
- 3 cups sliced fresh strawberries

Directions

1. Add the canola oil, egg whites and milk to mixing bowl and beat with a whisk.

2. In a separate bowl, mix together the flours, sugar and baking powder. Pour the sparkling water and the egg white mixture over the dry ingredients and mix until smooth.

3. Heat a Place a nonstick skillet over moderate heat. Then scoop 1/2 cup pancake batter into the heated skillet and cook until the top surface of the pancake is set and the bottom has browned, about 2-3 minutes.

4. Flip to cook the other side. Repeat this until all batter is gone.

5. Place the done pancakes into serving plates, garnish with strawberries and enjoy.

12. Healthy Tasty Breakfast

Prep time: 1 hour

Nutritional information per serving: Calories 321; Fat 10 g; Cholesterol 5 mg.

Serves 5.

Ingredients:

- 1 cup regular oats
- 1 cup plain low-fat yogurt
- 1 cup 1% low-fat milk
- 1/2 cup walnuts, coarsely chopped
- 1/3 cup honey
- 1/4 cup oat bran
- 3 tbs dried apricots, chopped
- 3 tbs dried figs, chopped
- 3 tbs pitted dates, chopped
- Raspberries or other fresh berries (optional)

Directions:

1. Place together the dried figs, dates, oat bran, dried apricots, walnuts, honey, regular oats in a large bowl.

2. Add the yogurt and milk and mix well to coat. Chill the mixture for 1-2 hours.

3. Place the muesli in a serving bowl, top with fresh berries and enjoy.

13. Rice Pudding

Prep time: 15 minutes

Cook time: 45 minutes

Nutritional information per serving: Calories 207; Fat 5 g; Cholesterol 8mg.

Serves 6

Ingredients:

- 1/2 cup basmati rice
- 4 cups milk
- 3 tablespoons sugar
- 1/4 cup raisins
- 1/2 tsp cardamom
- 1/4 tsp cinnamon
- 1/2 tsp rose water (optional)
- 1/4 almonds, chopped
- 1 tbs orange zest

Directions:

1. Add the rice to a pot of cold water and let sit for 10 minutes. Drain.
2. Combine the milk and sugar in a medium saucepan and bring to a simmer over medium-high heat.
3. Add the cinnamon, cardamom, raisins, give a stir. Slow down the heat, add the rice and let simmer, stirring often until thickened, about 40-45 minutes,
4. Add the rose water, if using, and remove the saucepan from the heat.

5. Ladle the pudding into serving bowls, garnish with orange zest and almonds and enjoy.

14. Banana, Strawberry and Honey Smoothie

Prep time: 10 minutes

Cook time: 0 minutes

Nutritional information per serving: Calories 159; Fat 0.22 g; Cholesterol 2 mg.

Serves 2

Ingredients

- 1 cup strawberries
- 1 tbs honey
- 1 tsp vanilla
- 1 cup fat free milk
- 1 banana

Directions

1. Combine the strawberries, honey, vanilla, banana and milk in a blender and pulse until smooth.
2. Pour the mixture into 2 serving glasses and enjoy.

Chapter 4 - Lunch Recipes

1. Chicken with Garlic, Basil, and Parsley

Prep time: 10 minutes

Cook time: 40 minutes

Nutritional information per serving: Calories 150; Fat 3.1 g; Cholesterol 67 mg.

Serves4.

Ingredients:

- 1 tbs dried parsley, divided
- 1 tbs dried basil, divided
- 4 skinless, boneless chicken breast halves
- 4 cloves garlic, thinly sliced
- 1/2 tsp salt
- 1/2 tsp red pepper flakes, crushed
- 2 tomatoes, sliced

Directions:

1. Preheat oven to 350 F (175 C). Lightly oil a 9x13 inch baking dish with cooking spray.

2. In a small cup, mix together 1 teaspoon of dried basil and 1 teaspoon of parsley and evenly coat the baking dish mixed spices.

3. Place the chicken breast halves in the prepared dish, and sprinkle with sliced garlic. Combine the remaining 2 teaspoons of basil, remaining 2 teaspoons parsley, red pepper and salt in a small cup and sprinkle over the chicken halves. Arrange tomato slices on the top, cover with a kitchen foil and transfer to the preheated oven.

4. Bake for about 25 minutes, then remove the cover, and let cook for another 15 minutes, or until the chicken is cooked through and golden brown.

2. Penne with Chicken and Asparagus

Prep time: 15 minutes

Cook time: 20 minutes

Nutritional information per serving: Calories 332, Fat 10.9 g, Cholesterol 20 mg.

Serves 8

Ingredients:

- 1 (16 oz./450 g) package dried penne pasta
- 5 tbs olive oil (divided)
- 2 skinless, boneless chicken breast halves (cut)
- salt and pepper (to taste)
- garlic powder (to taste)
- 1/2 cup low-sodium chicken broth
- 1 bunch slender asparagus spears (trimmed, cut)
- 1 clove garlic (thinly sliced)
- 1/4 cup Parmesan cheese

Directions:

1.   Place pasta in a pot of lightly salted boiling water and cook until al dente, about 8 to 10 minutes. Drain in the colander and set it aside.

2.   Add 3 tbs olive oil to a large saucepan and set over medium-high heat. Season the chicken with salt, pepper, and garlic powder and sauté in the pan until golden-brown on all sides, about 5 minutes. Transfer the chicken pieces to a plate lined with paper towels to drain.

3.   Add the chicken broth to the saucepan. Stir in the garlic, asparagus and a pinch more garlic powder, salt, and pepper and let steam, covered, until the asparagus has just softened, about 5 to 10

minutes. Return chicken back to the pan, and continue cooking until heated throughout.

4.   Add the chicken mixture to the pasta, and mix well to coat. Let the dish sit about 5 minutes. Drizzle the pasta mixture with 2 tablespoons of olive oil, sprinkle with Parmesan cheese and enjoy.

3. Black Beans and Rice

Prep time: 15 minutes

Cook time: 30 minutes

Nutritional information per serving: Calories 140 kcal, Fat 0.9 g, Cholesterol 0 mg,

Serves 10

Ingredients:

- 1 tsp olive oil
- 1 onion (chopped)
- 2 cloves garlic (minced)
- 3/4 cup white rice (uncooked)
- 1 1/2 cups low sodium, low fat vegetable broth
- 1 tsp ground cumin
- 1/4 tsp cayenne pepper
- 3 1/2 cups canned black beans(drained)

Directions:

1. Heat oil in a large saucepan over medium-high heat. Add the garlic and onion and fry for a couple of minutes, until tender. Then stir in the rice and sauté for 2-3 minutes.

2. Pour in the vegetable broth and bring to a boil. Then reduce the heat, put the lid on and cook for 20 minutes.

3. Add the black beans, season with cayenne pepper and cumin, give a stir and remove from heat. Let stand for 10 minutes before serving.

4. Oven Roasted Red Potatoes and Asparagus

Prep Time: 10 minutes
Cook Time: 40 minutes
Nutritional information per serving: Calories 149 kcal, Fat 4.9 g, Cholesterol 0 mg,

Serves 6

Ingredients:

- 1 1/2 lbs red potatoes (cut)
- 2 tbs extra virgin olive oil
- 8 cloves garlic (thinly sliced)
- 4 tsp rosemary (dried)
- 4 tsp thyme (dried)
- 2 tsp kosher salt
- 1 bunch fresh asparagus (trimmed, cut)
- ground black pepper (to taste)

Directions:

1. Preheat oven to 425 degrees F (220 degrees C).
2. Place the red potatoes in a large baking dish, sprinkle with thyme, garlic, rosemary and 1 tsp of kosher salt, add 1 tablespoon of olive oil and toss to coat.
3. Cover with aluminum foil and bake in the preheated oven for about 20 minutes. Then add the asparagus, remaining olive oil and salt. Cover, and let bake for another 15 minutes, until the potatoes have softened.
4. Increase the oven temperature to 450 degrees F (230 degrees C), remove the foil, and let cook for 5-10 minutes, until potatoes are golden brown.
5. Season with ground black pepper and serve.

5. Quinoa and Black Beans

Prep time: 15 minutes

Cook time: 35 minutes

Nutritional information per serving: Calories 153; Fat 1.7 g; Cholesterol 0 mg.

Serves 10.

Ingredients:

- 1 teaspoon vegetable oil
- 1 onion, chopped
- 3 cloves garlic, chopped
- 3/4 cup quinoa
- 1 1/2 cups vegetable broth
- 1 teaspoon ground cumin
- 1/4 teaspoon cayenne pepper
- Salt and ground black pepper to taste
- 1 cup frozen corn kernels
- 2 (15 ounce) cans black beans, rinsed and drained
- 1/2 cup fresh cilantro, chopped

Directions:

1. Add the oil to a large saucepan and set over moderate heat. Add the garlic and onion and sauté for 10 minutes, stirring frequently, until tender and lightly golden.

2. Add the quinoa; pour in the vegetable broth and let cook. Once it begins to boil, sprinkle with salt and pepper, and add the cumin and cayenne pepper.

3. Slow down the heat, put the lid on and let simmer until all liquid is absorbed and the quinoa has already softened, for 18-20 minutes.

4. Add the frozen corn, give a stir and let simmer for another 2-3 minutes until heated through.

5. Finally, stir in the black beans and chopped cilantro before removing the saucepan from the heat.

6. Mexican Rice

Prep time: 5 minutes

Cook time: 25 minutes

Nutritional information per serving: Calories 158; Fat 2.8 g; Cholesterol 1 mg.

Serves 6.

Ingredients:

- 1 cup long grain white rice
- 1 tbs vegetable oil
- 1 1/2 cups chicken broth
- 1/2 onion, finely chopped
- 1/2 green bell pepper, finely chopped
- 1 fresh jalapeno pepper, chopped
- 1 tomato, seeded and chopped
- 1 cube chicken bouillon
- Salt and pepper to taste
- 1/2 tsp ground cumin
- 1/2 cup fresh cilantro, chopped

Directions:

1. Add the oil to a medium saucepan and heat over medium heat. Stir in the rice and cook for 3-4 minutes.

2. Add the chicken broth. When it begins to a boil, add the green pepper, onion, sliced tomato, jalapeño and the bouillon cube.

3. Once the mixture returns to a boil, season with salt and pepper, sprinkle with garlic and cilantro and let simmer, covered, over low heat, about 20 minutes.

4. Place the rice in a serving plate and enjoy.

7. Spicy Pumpkin Soup

Prep time: 10 minutes

Cook time: 45 minutes

Nutritional information per serving: Calories 180; Fat 5 g; Cholesterol 5.4 mg.

Serves4

Ingredients:

- 2 lbs (900 g) pumpkin, peeled and seeded
- 2 tsp extra virgin olive oil
- 2 leeks, trimmed and sliced
- 1 garlic clove, crushed
- 1 tsp ginger, ground
- 1 tsp cumin, ground
- 3 cups vegetable stock or water
- Salt and pepper
- Coriander, chopped

Directions:

1. Peel the pumpkin and cut into coarse pieces. Add the oil to a large saucepan and set over medium heat. Add the garlic and leeks and cook until tender.

2. Stir in the cumin and ginger and cook for a minute. Add the pumpkin pieces; pour in the stock/water, sprinkle with salt and pepper and let cook over moderate heat.

3. Once boiling, reduce the heat to low and let simmer about 25-30 minutes, until the pumpkin has softened. Transfer the soup to a blender and pulse until puree.

4. Return back to the saucepan and heat for 1-2 minutes. Divide the soup among serving bowls, sprinkle with fresh chopped coriander and enjoy.

8. Lettuce-Wrap Tacos with Black Beans and Corn

Prep Time: 15 minutes
Nutritional information per serving: Calories: 170, Fat 6.5 g, Cholesterol 9mg.

Serves: 4

Ingredients:

- 1 cup canned no-salt-added black beans (rinsed ,drained)
- 1/2 cup frozen whole-kernel corn (thawed)
- 1 small Italian plum tomato (diced)
- 1/2 small avocado (diced)
- 2 tbs fresh cilantro (snipped)
- 1 tbs fresh lemon juice
- 1/2 tsp chili powder
- 8 Bibb lettuce leaves
- 1/2 cup low-fat Jack cheese (shredded)
- 1/2 cup salsa (lowest sodium available)

Directions:

1. Place the beans, tomato, corn, avocado, lemon juice, chili powder and cilantro in a small bowl and mix to combine.
2. Put 1/4 cup bean mixture into the middle of each lettuce leave. Top with the Jack cheese and salsa.
3. To make tacos, fold the edges of the lettuce leave over the filling.
4. To make burritos, roll the leave over the filling and tuck the ends in, securing each burrito with a toothpick.

9. Chicken and Black Bean Soup

Prep Time: 10 minutes

Cook Time: 26 minutes

Nutritional information: Calories 211, Fat 2.8g, Cholesterol 24mg.

Serves: 6-8

Ingredients:

- 2 tsp canola oil
- 1 medium onion (finely chopped)
- 1 medium carrot (chopped)
- 1/2 large red pepper
- 1 tsp cumin
- 1 tsp chili powder
- 2 (15-oz.) cans reduced sodium black beans (rinsed, drained)
- 3 cups fat-free, low-sodium chicken broth
- 1 (16-oz./450 g) jar mild salsa
- 1 1/2 cups skinless white-meat chicken (cooked, chopped)

Directions:

1. Add oil to a griddle and set over medium heat. Add the onions, peppers, carrots and sauté about 5 minutes.

2. Then stir in the chili powder and cumin and cook for another minute. Now pour in the broth, add black beans and salsa. Once boiled, put the lid on and let simmer for 15 minutes.

3. In the end, add the cooked chicken, let the soup simmer for another 5 minutes and remove the griddle from the heat.

4. Let stand for 5-10 minutes and enjoy.

10. Orecchiette with Broccoli Rabe & Chickpeas

Prep time: 10 minutes

Cook time: 20 minutes

Nutritional information per serving: Calories 410; Fat 9 g; Cholesterol 0 mg.

Serves 2.

Ingredients:

- 4 oz. (120 g) whole-wheat orecchiette (about 1 1/2 cups)
- 1/2 bunch broccoli rabe, ends trimmed and cut
- 3/4 cup vegetarian chicken-flavored broth
- 2 tsp all-purpose flour
- 1 tbs extra-virgin olive oil
- 4 large cloves garlic, minced
- 1/2 tsp minced fresh rosemary, or 1/8 teaspoon dried
- 1 8-oz. can chickpeas, drained and rinsed
- 2 tsp red-wine vinegar
- 1/8 tsp salt
- 1/4 tsp freshly ground pepper

Directions:

1. Add the pasta to a large pot of boiling water and set over medium-high heat. Let cook for 5-6 minutes.
2. Add the broccoli rabe and cook until the broccoli and pasta have just softened, 3-4 minutes.
3. Transfer to a colander to drain. Dry the pot as well.
4. In a small bowl, mix together the flour and broth.
5. Add the oil to the pot and set over moderate heat. Stir in the rosemary and garlic and sauté for 30-50 seconds.

6. Pour in the broth mixture and cook over low heat, stirring constantly, until the sauce has thickened.

7. Stir in the chickpeas and vinegar, season with salt and pepper. In the end add the pasta and broccoli and stir to coat. Cook for a couple of minutes until heated through.

11. Cod with Tomato Cream Sauce

Prep time: 15 minutes

Cook time: 20 minutes

Nutritional information per serving: Calories 227; Fat 10 g; Cholesterol 57 mg.

Serves 4.

Ingredients:

- 1-1 1/4 lbs cod (450-550 g) or tilapia fillets, cut into 4 pieces
- 3 tsp fresh thyme, chopped, divided
- 1/2 tsp salt, divided
- 1/4 tsp freshly ground pepper
- 1 tbs extra-virgin olive oil
- 1 shallot, chopped
- 2 cloves garlic, minced
- 3/4 cup white wine
- 1 (14-oz./400 g) can diced tomatoes
- 1/4 cup heavy cream or half-and-half
- 1/2 tsp cornstarch

Directions:

1. Sprinkle the fish fillets with 1/4 teaspoon salt, 1 teaspoon thyme, and pepper and let stand for 15 minutes.

2. Add the olive oil to a large frying and heat over medium heat. Add the garlic, shallot, and 1 teaspoon thyme and stir-fry until just tender, about 2-3 minutes.

3. Add the fish, tomatoes and wine and continue cooking. When it begins to bubble, reduce the heat, put the lid on and

let simmer until the fish flakes easily with a fork, about 5 minutes.

4. In a small bowl, combine the cornstarch and cream, stir in the remaining 1 teaspoon thyme and 1/4 teaspoon salt. Pour the mixture into the pan and cook for a minute, stirring constantly.

5. Place the fish in shallow bowls, spoon the sauce over the fish and serve.

12. Vegetable Soup

Prep time: 10 minutes

Cook time: 10 minutes

Nutritional information per serving: Calories 99; Fat 01 g; Cholesterol 0 mg.

Serves 8.

Ingredients:

- 3 medium zucchini, sliced
- 2 medium carrots, sliced
- 10 mushrooms, sliced
- 1 medium onion, sliced
- 1 10-oz. russet potato, peeled, cut into 1-inch pieces
- 3 14 1/2-ounce cans vegetable broth
- 3 cups canned tomatoes, crushed with added puree
- 1 14 1/2-ounce cans stewed tomatoes
- 3 tbs fresh parsley, chopped
- 2 tbs fresh cilantro, chopped
- 1 tbs chopped garlic
- 1 tsp dried basil

- 1 tsp dried oregano
- Additional fresh parsley, chopped

Directions:

1. Place the onion, garlic, carrots, mushrooms, stewed tomatoes, crushed tomatoes, zucchini and potato in a large griddle and set over moderate heat.

2. Pour in the vegetable broth; add 3 tablespoons parsley, cilantro, basil and oregano. When it begins to boil, slow down the heat, put the lid on and let simmer until vegetables are soft, about 25 minutes.

3. Transfer the cooking liquid to a large pot, reserving the vegetables. Put 3 cups vegetables in a blender, add ¼ cup cooking liquid and pulse until puree. Add this mixture to the pot of cooking liquid; add the remaining vegetables to the soup. Season the soup with salt and pepper. Let simmer for 5 minutes and then return off the heat.

4. Divide the soup among serving bowls, sprinkle with chopped parsley and enjoy.

13. Roasted Veggie Pitas

Prep time: 5 minutes

Cook time: 15 minutes

Nutritional information per serving: Calories 270; Fat 16 g; Cholesterol 16 mg.

Serves 4.

Ingredients:

- 1 small zucchini thinly sliced lengthwise
- 1 small yellow summer squash thinly sliced lengthwise
- 1 medium onion, thinly sliced
- 1/2 cup sliced fresh mushrooms
- 1/2 of a red sweet pepper, cut into thin strips
- 2 tbs olive oil
- 1/2 tsp salt
- 1/4 tsp ground black pepper
- 2 large pita bread rounds, halved
- 4 tsp bottled vinaigrette or Italian salad dressing
- 3/4 cup smoked provolone or mozzarella cheese, shredded

Directions:

1. Preheat oven to 450°F (220 °C).
2. Combine the sliced summer squash, zucchini, mushrooms, sweet pepper and onion in a large bowl.
3. Add the oil, season with salt and black pepper and mix to combine. Transfer the vegetable mixture to a baking pan and spread evenly.

4. Roast in the oven for 9- 10 minutes or until vegetables have softened.

5. Fill the roasted vegetables into pita pockets, sprinkle with cheese, and drizzle with Italian salad dressing.

6. Bake the pita sandwiches in the oven for 2-3 minutes, until heated through and the cheese is melted.

14. Florentine Ravioli

Prep time: 5 minutes

Cook time: 17 minutes

Nutritional information per serving: Calories 263; Fat 13 g; Cholesterol 28 mg.

Serves 4.

Ingredients:

- 1 20-oz. (550 g) package frozen cheese ravioli, or tortellini (4 cups)
- 6 tsp extra-virgin olive oil, divided
- 4 cloves garlic, minced
- 1/4 tsp salt
- 1/8-1/4 tsp crushed red pepper
- 1 (16-oz./450 g) bag frozen chopped or whole-leaf spinach
- 1/2 cup water
- 1/4 cup Parmesan cheese, freshly grated

Directions:

1. Place ravioli in a large pot of boiling water and cook following the package instructions.
2. Add 2 teaspoons of olive oil to a large frying pan and heat over medium heat.
3. Add the garlic and stir-fry until fragrant, about 40 seconds. Add the spinach, water, season with salt and crushed red pepper to taste and cook, until the spinach wilts, stirring often, about 6-7 minutes.
4. Place the spinach into 4 bowls, add the pasta and drizzle with the remaining oil. Sprinkle with grated Parmesan and serve immediately.

15. Pizza Naturale

Prep time: 30 minutes

Cook time: 30 minutes

Nutritional information per serving: Calories 129.9; Fat 13 g; Cholesterol 21mg.

Serves 12

Ingredients:

- 3 tbs extra virgin olive oil
- 1 homemade pizza dough
- 4 cups sweet onions, thinly sliced
- 3 garlic cloves, minced
- 3 cups mushrooms (sliced)
- 8 oz.(225gr.) Mozzarella cheese, thinly sliced
- Salt and pepper
- Fresh parsley, chopped
- 2 tsp fresh rosemary, chopped

Directions:

1. Preheat oven to 375°F (190C)

2. Lay prepared pizza dough in a baking tray or a round pizza sheet. Top with cheese slices.

3. In a large skillet, heat 2 tablespoons olive oil and sauté onions, covered, stirring occasionally, over medium low heat for 13-15 minutes. Once the onions are tender, remove the cover and let cook over medium heat for another 5-10 minutes longer or until onions brown.

4. Transfer the onions to a bowl and set aside.

5. In the same skillet, place mushrooms, remaining 1 tablespoon olive oil, garlic, and rosemary. Sauté over medium heat until mushrooms are tender and lightly brown; drain well.

6. Pour mushroom mixture over cheese. Spoon the onions over top of the pizza.

7. Bake in the preheated oven at 375°F (190C) for 25-30 minutes or until the edges of pizza are slightly crisp and brown.

8. Remove from the oven, season with salt and pepper to taste and let stand for 5 minutes. Garnish with parsley. Cut the pizza into square pieces and serve immediately. Enjoy!

16. Tabbouleh with Feta and Sweet Soybeans

Prep time: 15 minutes

Cook time: 35 minutes

Nutritional information per serving: Calories 320; Fat 10 g; Cholesterol 8 mg.

Serves 6.

Ingredients:

- 2 1/2 cups water
- 1 1/4 cups bulgur
- 1/4 cup lemon juice
- 3 tbs purchased basil pesto
- 2 cups fresh or thawed frozen shelled sweet soybeans (edamame)
- 2 cups cherry tomatoes, cut up
- 1/3 cup crumbled feta cheese
- 1/3 cup green onions, thinly sliced
- 2 tbs snipped fresh parsley
- 1/4 tsp ground black pepper
- Fresh parsley sprigs (optional)

Directions:

1. Add the water to a medium pot and set over high heat. When it begins to boil, add the bulgur and return to a boil.

2. Slow down the heat, put the lid on and let simmer, until all water is almost absorbed. Transfer the bulgur to a large salad bowl

3. Combine the pesto and lemon juice in a small bowl and pour over the bulgur. Add the cherry tomatoes, soybeans, green

onions, parsley and feta cheese, season with pepper and mix well to combine.

4. Garnish the salad with parsley sprigs, if using and enjoy.

16. Barley - Vegetable Chicken Soup

Prep time: 10 minutes

Cook time: 45 minutes

Nutritional information per serving: Calories 137; Fat 1 g; Cholesterol 33 mg.

Serves 8.

Ingredients:

- 8 cups reduced-sodium chicken broth
- 1/2 cup regular barley
- 4 skinless, boneless chicken breast halves (1 to 1 1/4 pounds total), cut into 3/4-inch cubes
- 3 stalks celery, sliced
- 3 medium carrots, sliced
- 1 medium onion, chopped
- 1/4 cup snipped fresh parsley or 2 tablespoons dried parsley flakes
- 1 tbs snipped fresh sage or rosemary or 1 teaspoon dried sage or rosemary, crushed
- 1/4 tsp ground black pepper
- 1 cup green, yellow, and/or red sweet pepper, chopped
- Parsley (optional)

Directions:

1. Add the broth to a large saucepan and bring to a boil over medium-high heat.
2. Add the barley, slow down the heat and let simmer, covered, for 25 minutes.

3. Stir in the carrots, chicken, dried parsley, celery, sage, onion, season with black pepper and return the soup to a boil. Put the lid on and let simmer for about 8-10 minutes. Stir in the sweet pepper and cook for another 5 minutes until vegetables are soft and chicken is almost cooked through.

4. Sprinkle with fresh chopped parsley and remove from the heat. Let stand, covered, for 15 minutes before serving.

17. Eggplant Pomodoro Pasta

Prep time: 10 minutes

Cook time: 20 minutes

Nutritional information per serving: Calories 282; Fat 7 g; Cholesterol 0 mg.

Serves 6.

Ingredients:

- 2 tbs extra-virgin olive oil
- 1 medium eggplant, cut into cubes
- 2 cloves garlic, minced
- 4 plum tomatoes, diced
- 1/3 cup pitted green olives, chopped
- 2 tbs red-wine vinegar
- 4 tsp capers, rinsed
- 3/4 tsp salt
- 1/2 tsp freshly ground pepper
- 1/4 tsp crushed red pepper, (optional)
- 12 oz. (340 g) whole-wheat angel hair pasta
- 1/4 cup fresh parsley, or basil, chopped

Directions:

1. In a large frying pan, heat the oil over medium heat. Add the eggplant and cook, stirring occasionally, until just tender, about 4-5 minutes.

2. Add the garlic and cook, until lightly brown and fragrant, about 1 minute. Then add the olives, capers, tomatoes.

3. Add the vinegar and season with salt, pepper and crushed red pepper (if using). Continue cooking, until the tomatoes start to break down, stirring frequently, 6-7 minutes more.

4. Meanwhile, add the pasta to a pot of boiling water and cook following the package instructions, about 6 minutes. Drain in a colander.

5. Place the cooked pasta in a serving dish, add the tomato sauce on the top, garnish parsley or basil and enjoy.

18. Salmon with Wilted Greens

Prep time: 15 minutes

Cook time: 35 minutes

Nutritional information per serving: Calories 256; Fat 9g; Cholesterol 31 mg.

Serves 4.

Ingredients:

- 4 6 - ounces fresh or frozen salmon steaks, cut 1-inch thick
- 3 tbs orange juice concentrate
- 2 tbs light soy sauce
- 1 tbsp honey
- 2 tsp cooking oil
- 1 tsp toasted sesame oil
- 1/2 teaspoon grated fresh ginger or 1/4 teaspoon ground ginger
- 6 cups torn mixed greens (such as spinach, Swiss chard, mustard, beet, or collard greens)
- 1 medium orange, peeled and sectioned
- 1 small red sweet pepper, cut into thin strips

Directions:

1. Wash the fish in cold water and pat dry.
2. Make the dressing by combining soy sauce, honey, concentrate, sesame oil, cooking oil, 3 tablespoons water, orange juice and ginger in a small bowl.
3. Lightly coat the rack of a broiler pan with oil and place the fish on it. Broil for 4-5 minutes per side. Flip with a spatula to brown the other side.

4. Spoon 1 tablespoon of the dressing over the fish and let broil for 5-6 minutes until the fish is opaque throughout.

5. In a large bowl combine the sliced orange and greens. Add the remaining dressing to a large frying pan and put over high heat.

6. Stir in the red pepper strips. Cook for a few seconds. Pour the hot dressing over the greens and toss to coat.

7. Divide the greens among 4 serving plates. Put a salmon steak on the top and serve.

19. Sesame Orange Beef

Prep time: 15 minutes

Cook time: 35 minutes

Nutritional information per serving: Calories 348; Fat 7 g; Cholesterol 52 mg.

Serves 4.

Ingredients

- 8 oz. (240 g)fresh green beans, halved crosswise
- 2 teaspoons sesame seeds
- 1/2 cup orange juice
- 2 tbs reduced-sodium soy sauce
- 1 tbs toasted sesame oil
- 1 tsp cornstarch
- 1/2 teaspoon finely shredded orange peel
- Cooking spray
- 1/2 cup bias-sliced green onions
- 1 tbs grated fresh ginger
- 2 cloves garlic, minced
- 1 tsp cooking oil
- 12 oz. (340 g) boneless beef sirloin steak, thinly sliced
- 2 cups hot cooked brown rice
- 2 oranges, peeled, thinly sliced crosswise

Directions

1. Add little water to a medium pot and bring to a boil. Add the green beans and cook for 7-8 minutes until tender. Drain in a colander and set aside.

2. Place the sesame seeds in a small pan and cook over moderate heat, until toasted, about 2 minutes.

3. In a small bowl, whisk together the sesame oil, soy sauce, cornstarch, orange peel and orange juice; set aside.

4. Lightly oil the pan with a cooking spray and place over medium- high heat.

5. Add the garlic, green onions and, ginger to the hot pan and sauté for a minute. Stir in the green beans, cook for 2-4 minutes and remove the vegetables from the pan.

6. Add the oil to the hot pan and set over medium-high heat. Add the beef and cook for 3-5 minutes until lightly golden.

7. Add the sauce to the pan and cook for about 3 minutes until thickened. Add the vegetables and the meat and cook for a few minutes until heated through.

8. Serve the dish over noodles or hot cooked brown rice. Top with orange sections and sprinkle with toasted sesame seeds.

20. Healthy Green Salad with Toasted Pecans and Honey

Prep Time: 10 minutes

Cook Time: 10 minutes

Nutritional information per serving: Calories 225,Fat 18 g,Cholesterol 0 mg.

Serves 2

Ingredients:

- 1 tsp sherry vinegar
- 1 tsp honey
- 1/4 tsp Dijon mustard
- 1 tbs olive oil
- 1 tbs minced shallots
- 1/4 tsp kosher salt
- 1/4 tsp freshly ground black pepper
- 2 cups escarole, chopped
- 2 cups romaine lettuce, chopped
- 1 cup pitted prunes, chopped
- 1/4 cup pecans, toasted, chopped

Preparation

1. In a small bowl, whisk together the Dijon mustard, honey and sherry vinegar.

2. Then add the olive oil in a slow steam and mix to coat. Stir in the shallots, season with salt and fresh black pepper; set aside.

3. In a large bowl, place together the romaine lettuce and escarole. Add the pecans, and prunes and gently toss to combine.

4. Add the honey dressing to the salad and mix to coat. Serve immediately.

21. Spinach with Garbanzo Beans

Prep time: 15 minutes

Cook time: 10 minutes

Nutritional information per serving: Calories 169; Fat 4.9 g; Cholesterol 0 mg.

Serves 4

Ingredients:

- 1 tbs extra-virgin olive oil
- 4 cloves garlic, minced
- 1/2 onion, diced
- 1 (10 oz./280 g) box frozen chopped spinach, thawed and drained well
- 1 (12 oz./340 g) can garbanzo beans, drained
- 1/2 tsp cumin
- 1/2 tsp salt

Directions:

1. Add the olive oil to a medium frying pan and heat over medium-low heat. Add the onion and garlic to the pan and sauté until soft and lightly golden, 5-7 minutes.

2. Add the garbanzo beans, spinach, season with salt and cumin. During cooking slightly mash the beans with a spoon. Let cook for a couple of minutes until heated through. Great to be served with rice or noodles.

Chapter 5 - Dinner Recipes

1. Chicken & Spinach Soup with Fresh Pesto

Prep time: 10 minutes

Cook time: 20 minutes

Nutritional information per serving: Calories 204; Fat 8 g ,
Cholesterol 29 mg ;
Serves 5

Ingredients:

- 2 tsp plus 1 tbs extra-virgin olive oil (divided)
- 1/2 cup carrot or diced red bell pepper
- 1 large boneless, skinless chicken breast (cut)
- 1 large clove garlic (minced)
- 5 cups reduced-sodium chicken broth
- 1 1/2 teaspoons marjoram (dried)
- 6 oz. baby spinach (coarsely chopped)
- 1 (15-oz.) can cannellini beans (rinsed)
- 1/4 cup Parmesan cheese (grated)
- 1/3 cup lightly packed fresh basil leaves
- Freshly ground pepper (to taste)
- 3/4 cup plain or herbed multigrain croutons for garnish (optional)

Directions:

1. Add 2 tsp oil to a large soup pot and set over medium-high heat. Add the chicken and carrot (or bell pepper) and sauté for 3-4 minutes, turning the chicken and stirring frequently,

    until the chicken acquires golden crust. Stir in the garlic and stir-fry, for about a minute.

2. Now add the marjoram, pour in the broth and bring the soup to a boil over high heat. Reduce the heat and let the soup simmer, stirring occasionally, until the chicken is cooked through, about 5 minutes.

3. Transfer the cooked chicken pieces to a cutting board using a slotted spoon and let cool. Stir in the beans and spinach to the soup pot and let cook for 5 minutes.

4. Add the remaining 1 tbs oil, basil and Parmesan to a mini food processor, add a little water and pulse until a coarse paste has formed, scraping down the sides as necessary.

5. Cut the chicken into small pieces and add to the soup. Stir in also the pesto, season with pepper and cook until heated through, 1-2 minutes.

6. Ladle the soup into serving bowls, garnish with croutons and enjoy.

2. Grilled Salmon & Zucchini with Red Pepper Sauce

Prep time: 25 minutes

Cook time: 10 minutes

Nutritional information per serving: Calories 280; Fat 13 g; Cholesterol 66 mg.

Serves 4

Ingredients:

- 1/3 cup almonds (toasted, sliced)
- 1/4 cup jarred roasted red peppers (chopped)
- 1/4 cup grape tomatoes or cherry tomatoes (halved)
- 1 small clove garlic
- 1 tbs extra-virgin olive oil
- 1 tbs sherry vinegar or red-wine vinegar
- 1 tsp paprika (preferably smoked)
- 3/4 tsp salt (divided)
- 1/2 tsp freshly ground pepper (divided)
- 1 1/4 lbs (570 g) salmon fillet (skinned, cut into 4 portions)
- 2 medium zucchini or summer squash (halved)
- Canola or olive oil cooking spray
- 1 tbs fresh parsley (chopped, for garnish)

Directions:

1. Preheat grill to medium.
2. Place tomatoes, garlic, almonds, vinegar, peppers, oil, paprika, 1/4 tsp salt and 1/4 tsp pepper in a food processor or blender and pulse until smooth; set aside.

3. Sprinkle zucchini and salmon with cooking spray, then season with the remaining 1/2 tsp salt and 1/4 tsp pepper and grill, turning once, until the salmon is cooked through and the zucchini is golden and tender, about 3 minutes each side.

4. Transfer the zucchini to a cutting board and let cool. Then thinly slice it and place in a bowl. Pour half of the prepared sauce over the zucchini. Divide the mixture among 4 serving plates. Place alongside a piece of grilled salmon, top with a little of the remaining sauce. Decorate the dish with parsley and enjoy.

3. Black Bean and Tortilla Bake

Prep Time: 5 minutes

Cook Time: 30 minutes

Nutritional information per serving: Calories 270, Fat 4.6 g, Cholesterol 8 mg.

Serves 6.

Ingredients:

- 1 garlic clove, minced
- 1/2 cup onion, chopped
- 1 cup tomato, chopped
- 1/2 cup chopped green onion
- 1/2 tsp chili powder
- 2 tsp cumin powder
- 1 (8 oz./ 225 g) can tomato sauce
- 1 (16 oz./ 450 g) can black beans, rinsed and drained
- 1 tbs cilantro, chopped
- Salt and pepper
- 12 soft corn tortillas
- 8 oz. (225 g) low-fat cheddar cheese, shredded (reserve 2 tablespoons)

Directions:

1. Preheat oven to 350 °F (175 °C). Coat a large frying pan with cooking spray and set over moderate heat.
2. Stir in the onions, garlic, tomato, green onion, chili powder and cumin and sauté until the onions have softened.
3. Stir in the tomato sauce and cook for another 5 minutes.

4. Add the beans, cilantro, season with salt and pepper and stir to combine.

5. Coat a baking dish with cooking spray.

6. Place 4 tortillas in the baking dish, top with 1/3 of the bean mixture and 1/3 cheese. Repeat the process 2 more times. Sprinkle the reserved 2 tbs of cheese over the top and transfer to the oven. Cover with foil and bake for about 20 minutes, then remove the cover and bake for another 10 minutes.

7. Remove from the oven and let cool for about 10 minutes.

8. Cut into squares and serve.

4. Creamy Hungarian Mushroom Soup

Prep time: 15 minutes

Cook time: 25 minutes

Nutritional information per serving: Calories 232; Fat 6 g; Cholesterol 37 mg.

Serves 6

Ingredients:

- 1 tbs extra-virgin olive oil
- 1 1/2 pounds mushrooms (thinly sliced)
- 1 medium onion (diced)
- 3 tbs all-purpose flour
- 2 tbs paprika
- 2 tbs dried dill
- 4 cups mushroom broth or reduced-sodium beef broth
- 2 cups low-fat milk
- 1 1/2 pounds russet potatoes (peeled, cut)
- 1/2 cup reduced-fat sour cream
- 3/4 tsp salt

Directions:

1. Add oil to a large saucepan and heat over medium-high heat. Add onion and mushrooms and sauté about 10-15 minutes, stirring occasionally, until most of the liquid evaporates.

2. Slow down the heat to medium and cook for another 3-4 minutes until the mushrooms are tender, stirring frequently. Stir in the flour, season with dill and paprika and cook for a few seconds, stirring constantly.

3. Now add the milk, broth and potatoes; cover and bring to a simmer. Reduce the heat, remove the lid and let simmer, until the potatoes are soft, about 5 minutes. Remove the soup from the heat, stir in sour cream, season with salt and serve.

5. Chunky Minestrone Soup

Prep Time: 15 minutes
Cook Time: 30 minutes
Nutritional information per serving: Calories 296.5, Fat 3.2 g, Cholesterol 0.0.

Serves 6-8

Ingredients:

- 3 large carrots (roughly chopped)
- 1 large onion (roughly chopped)
- 4 celery ribs (roughly chopped)
- 1 tbs olive oil
- 2 garlic cloves (crushed)
- 2 large potatoes (cut)
- 2 tbs tomato paste
- 8 cups vegetable broth
- salt and pepper
- 14 oz.(400 g) tomatoes (chopped)
- 14 oz. (400 g) cannellini beans (drained)
- 5 oz.(140 g) spaghetti (snapped into short lengths)
- Savoy cabbage (shredded)

Directions:

1. Place the onion, carrots and celery in a food processor or blender and process until finely chopped.
2. Add the oil to a skillet and heat over moderate heat. Add the garlic, chopped vegetables and potatoes and sauté for 5 minutes until tender.

3. Add the tomato paste, tomatoes and broth and bring the soup to a boil, then reduce the heat, put the lid on and let simmer, for 10 minutes.
4. Now stir in the pasta and the beans and cook for 7-8 minutes, then add the cabbage and cook for another 2-3 minutes
5. Adjust seasonings to taste and serve with crusty bread.

6. Tuna Pasta with Olives & Artichokes

Prep time: 15 minutes

Cook time: 25 minutes

Nutritional information per serving: Calories 421; Fat 17 g, Cholesterol 26 mg;
Serves 4

Ingredients:

- 8 oz. (230 g) tuna steak (cut into 3 pieces)
- 4 tbs extra-virgin olive oil, divided
- 2 tsp lemon zest (freshly grated)
- 2 tsp chopped fresh rosemary or 1 teaspoon dried (divided)
- 1/2 tsp salt (divided)
- 1/4 tsp freshly ground pepper
- 6 oz. (170 g) whole-wheat rotini or penne pasta
- 1 (10-oz./280 g) package frozen artichoke hearts (thawed, squeezed dry)
- 1/4 cup green olives (chopped)
- 3 cloves garlic (minced)
- 2 cups grape tomatoes (halved)
- 1/2 cup white wine
- 2 tbs lemon juice
- 1/4 cup fresh basil or parsley (chopped, for garnish)

Directions:

1. Preheat grill to medium-high.
2. Place the fish in a bowl; add lemon zest, 1 tbs of oil, 1 tsp fresh rosemary (or 1/2 tsp dried), 1/4 tsp salt and pepper. Toss well to coat.

3. Grill the tuna about 3 minutes per side, until cooked through. Transfer to a plate and let cool. Then flake the tuna into small pieces.

4. Meanwhile, put pasta in a pot of boiling water and cook following the package instructions. Transfer to the colander to drain.

5. Add the remaining 3 tbs of oil to a large pan and heat over medium heat. Stir in the garlic, olives, artichoke hearts and the remaining rosemary and sauté for a couple of minutes, stirring frequently, until the garlic is just brown.

6. Add tomatoes and wine and bring the mixture to a boil, stirring occasionally, and let cook about 3 minutes.

7. Then stir in the tuna, pasta, lemon juice, the remaining 1/4 tsp salt and cook for 2 minutes, until heated through.

8. Place the pasta in a serving plate, sprinkle with chopped basil (or parsley) and serve.

7. Almond-&-Lemon-Crusted Fish with Spinach

Prep time: 5 minutes

Cook time: 5 minutes

Nutritional information per serving: Calories 249; Fat 13 g; Cholesterol 46 mg.

Serves 4.

Ingredients:

- Zest and juice of 1 lemon, divided
- 1/2 cup sliced almonds, coarsely chopped
- 1 tbs finely chopped fresh dill or 1 teaspoon dried
- 1 tbs plus 2 teaspoons extra-virgin olive oil, divided
- 1 tsp kosher salt, divided
- Freshly ground pepper to taste
- 1 1/4 lbs (566 g) cod or halibut, cut into 4 portions
- 4 tsp Dijon mustard
- 2 cloves garlic, slivered
- 1 pound baby spinach
- Lemon wedges for garnish

Directions:

1. Preheat oven to 400°F (200 °C). Coat a rimmed baking sheet with cooking spray.

2. Combine lemon zest, almonds, dill, 1 tablespoon oil, 1/2 teaspoon salt and pepper in a small bowl. Place fish on the prepared baking sheet and spread each portion with 1 teaspoon mustard. Divide the almond mixture among the portions, pressing it onto the mustard.

3. Bake the fish until opaque in the center, about 7 to 9 minutes, depending on thickness.

4. Meanwhile, heat the remaining 2 teaspoons oil in a Dutch oven over medium heat. Add garlic and cook, stirring, until fragrant but not brown, about 30 seconds. Stir in spinach, lemon juice and the remaining 1/2 teaspoon salt; season with pepper. Cook, stirring often, until the spinach is just wilted, 2 to 4 minutes. Cover to keep warm. Serve the fish with the spinach and lemon wedges, if desired.

8. Black Bean & Salmon Tostadas

Prep time: 10 minutes

Cook time: 15 minutes

Nutritional information per serving: Calories 319; Fat 11 g; Cholesterol 16 mg.

Serves 4.

Ingredients:

- 8 6-inch corn tortillas
- Canola oil cooking spray
- 1 6- to 7-ounce can boneless, skinless wild Alaskan salmon, drained
- 1 avocado, diced
- 2 tbs minced pickled jalapeños, plus 2 tablespoons pickling juice from the jar, divided
- 2 cups coleslaw mix or shredded cabbage
- 2 tbs cilantro, chopped
- 1 15-ounce can black beans, rinsed
- 3 tbs reduced-fat sour cream
- 2 tbs prepared salsa
- 2 scallions, chopped
- Lime wedges (optional)

Directions:

1. Preheat oven to 375°F (190 °C) and set racks in lower and upper thirds of the oven.

2. Brush both sides of the tortillas with cooking spray, put on 2 separate baking sheets and bake in the oven, flipping once, until light golden, about 15 minutes.

3. In a bowl place together the jalapeños, avocado and salmon.

4. In a separate bowl, combine the cabbage, pickling juice and cilantro.

5. In a blender, combine the sour cream, black beans, scallions and salsa and pulse until smooth. Pour the mixture in a microwave-safe bowl and heat on HIGH about 2 minutes.

6. Spoon some bean mixture onto each tortilla and spread evenly. Top with some salmon mixture and cabbage salad. Great to serve with lime wedges.

9. Chicken Stew

Prep Time: 10 minutes

Cook Time: 30 minutes

Nutritional information per serving: Calories 208, Fat 6 g, Cholesterol 42mg.

Serves 6.

Ingredients

- 5 tsp extra-virgin olive oil, divided
- 1 lb (450 g) chicken tenders, cut into bite-size pieces
- 1 large onion, chopped
- 4 medium parsnips, peeled and chopped
- 2 medium carrots, peeled and chopped
- 2 tsp chopped fresh rosemary or 1/2 teaspoon dried
- 1/2 tsp salt
- 1/4 tsp freshly ground pepper
- 4 cups reduced-sodium chicken broth
- 2 Granny Smith apples, peeled and chopped
- 2 tsp cider vinegar

Directions:

1. Add 2 teaspoons of olive oil to a griddle and heat over medium heat.

2. Add the chicken and sauté, turning occasionally, until just cooked through, about 5 minutes. Remove from the heat and set aside.

3. Add the remaining 3 teaspoons of oil to a large saucepan and set over medium heat. Add the carrots, onion, parsnips, rosemary, sprinkle with salt and pepper and cook, stirring

frequently, until the vegetables are just tender, about 5 minutes.

4. Add the apples and broth and bring to a boil over medium-high heat.

5. Slow down the heat and let simmer stirring frequently, until the vegetables are soft, 9- 10 minutes.

6. Add the chicken and vinegar, cook for another 2-3 minutes and remove from the heat.

7. Ladle the stew into soup bowls and serve immediately.

10. Healthy Bean Soup with Kale

Prep Time: 2 minutes

Cook Time: 20 minutes

Nutritional information per serving: Calories 214.6, Fat 3.8 g, Cholesterol 0 mg.

Serves 8.

Ingredients:

- 1 tbs olive oil
- 8 garlic cloves, minced
- 1 medium yellow onion, chopped
- 4 cups raw kale, chopped
- 4 cups chicken broth or 4 cups vegetable broth, divided
- 2 (15 ounce) cans cannellini or navy beans, undrained, split
- 2 (15 ounce) cans sliced carrots, undrained
- 1 (28 ounce) can diced tomatoes
- 2 tsp Italian herb seasoning
- Salt and pepper
- 1 cup parsley, chopped
- Parmesan cheese, shredded

Directions:

1. Add the olive oil to a large saucepan and set over medium heat. Add the onion and garlic and sauté for a few minutes until tender and lightly golden.

2. Rinse the kale and pat to drain. Add the kale to the saucepan and stir-fry until wilted, about 10-12 minutes.

3. Add the tomatoes, carrots, herbs, 2 cups of the beans, reserving 1 cup, pour in 3 cups of the broth, reserving 1 cup,

season with salt and pepper. Stir and let simmer for about 5 minutes.

4. Place the reserved beans and broth in a blender and process until puree.

5. Pour the mixture into the soup to thicken it and continue cooking for another 15 minutes.

6. Divide the soup among serving bowls, sprinkle with shredded cheese and chopped parsley.

7. Enjoy.

11. Parmesan and Root Vegetable Lasagna

Prep time: 5 minutes

Cook time: 15 minutes

Nutritional information per serving: Calories 320; Fat 7g; Cholesterol 19mg.

Serves 10.

Ingredients:

- 6 cups (about 2 1/2 lbs/1200 g) butternut squash, peeled, cubed
- 2 1/4 (1lb/450 g) cups sweet potato, peeled, cubed
- 2 cups onion, coarsely chopped, divided
- 1 tablespoon olive oil
- Cooking spray
- 4 cups 1% low-fat milk
- 1/8 tsp ground nutmeg
- 1/8 tsp ground cinnamon
- 1 bay leaf
- 1/3 cup all-purpose flour (about)
- 1/2 tsp salt
- 1/4 tsp freshly ground black pepper
- 1 1/4 cups (5 oz./150 g) Parmigiano - Reggiano cheese, grated
- 9 packaged no-boil lasagna noodles
- 1 1/2 cups (6 ounces) shredded part-skim mozzarella cheese

Directions:

1. Preheat oven to 450°F (220 °C).

2. Coat a baking dish with cooking spray. Add the potato, oil, squash and 1 cup chopped onion to the prepared dish, mix to coat vegetables with oil. Bake in the oven for 25-30 minutes or until vegetables have softened, set aside.

3. In a medium pot, place together the milk, cinnamon, nutmeg, bay leaf and the remaining 1 cup onion and place over medium-high heat. Once boiling, reduce the heat, let simmer for 2-3 minutes and turn off the heat. Let stand 10-15 minutes.

4. Using a fine sieve, strain the milk mixture and return back to the pot. Whisk in the flour, salt and pepper and cook the mixture over moderate heat for 10 minutes, stirring often until it is thickened. Add the grated cheese and remove the milk mixture from heat.

5. Preheat oven to 375°F (175 °C).

6. Coat a baking pan with cooking spray. Add the mixture to the baking pan and spread evenly. Place 3 noodles over the mixture. Spoon half of the squash mixture, 1/2 cup mozzarella and 1 cup milk mixture on the noodles. Alternately repeat this for the remaining 3 noodles.

7. Once you have put the last 3 noodles, cover with milk mixture and sprinkle with 1/2 cup mozzarella. Cover the lasagna with foil and bake in the oven for 25-30 minutes.

8. Remove the foil and bake for another 20 minutes. Let cool for 15 minutes and serve.

12. Cashew Chicken

Prep Time: 1 hr 15 minutes
Cook Time:20 minutes
Nutritional information per serving: Calories 311,Fat 5 g,Cholesterol 44 mg.

Serves 6

Ingredients:

- 1 lb (450 g) skinless, boneless chicken breasts, cut into strips
- 1/4 cup orange juice
- 1 tbs plus 1 teaspoon cornstarch, divided
- 1 tsp vegetable oil
- 1/4 cup chopped cashews
- 1 (8-ounce) can sliced water chestnuts, drained
- 1 cup green bell pepper, chopped (about 1 large)
- 1/2 cup green onions, chopped (about 2)
- 1 tbs fresh ginger, minced
- 1 cup fat-free, less-sodium chicken broth
- 2 tbs low-sodium soy sauce
- 1 (11-ounce) can mandarin oranges in light syrup, drained
- 3 cups hot cooked brown rice

Directions:

1. Place the chicken strips, 1 teaspoon cornstarch and orange juice in a medium bowl, put the lid on and refrigerate for 1 hour.
2. Add the vegetable oil to a nonstick frying pan and set over medium heat.
3. Add the cashews and stir-fry for 40 seconds.

4. Remove from the pan and set aside. Add the marinated chicken to the pan and cook over medium-high heat, uncovered, about 10 minutes or until chicken is lightly golden, stirring frequently.

5. Stir in the water chestnuts, onions, ginger, season with pepper and let cook for 5 minutes.

6. In a small bowl, whisk the soy sauce, broth and 1 tablespoon cornstarch and add to the pan.

7. Once it begins to boil, slow down the heat, and cook, stirring constantly, until the mixture thickens.

8. Stir in the oranges and remove from the heat. Place the rice in a serving plate, top with chicken mixture.

9. Garnish the dish with cashews and serve immediately.

13. Chili Bean-Stuffed Peppers

Prep time: 5 minutes

Cook time: 6 ½ hrs

Nutritional information per serving: Calories 283; Fat 8g; Cholesterol 19mg.

Serves 4.

Ingredients:

- 4 medium green, red, or yellow sweet peppers
- 1 cup cooked rice
- 1 15 oz. can chili beans with chili gravy
- 1 15 oz. can no-salt-added tomato sauce
- 1/3 cup onion, finely chopped
- 3 oz. (90 g) Monterey Jack cheese, shredded (3/4 cup)

Directions:

1. Trim the peppers, cut the tops and membranes, and gently remove the seeds. Thinly chop the tops and set aside.

2. Place the beans and rice in medium bowl and mix well. Fill the mixture into the peppers. Add the tomato sauce to the slow cooker, mix in the onion and chopped pepper. Put the peppers stuffed side up in a slow cooker.

3. Put the lid on and cook over low heat for about 6 ½ hours.

4. Place the cooked peppers on a serving plate, top with tomato sauce and shredded cheese.

5. Enjoy.

14. Tasty Sesame Noodles

Prep time: 10 minutes

Cook time: 10 minutes

Nutritional information per serving: Calories 345; Fat 12 g; Cholesterol 0 mg.

Serves 8.

Ingredients

- 1 lb (450 g) whole-wheat spaghetti
- 1/2 cup reduced-sodium soy sauce
- 2 tbs sesame oil
- 2 tbs canola oil
- 2 tbs rice-wine vinegar, or lime juice
- 1 1/2 tsp crushed red pepper
- 1 bunch scallions, sliced, divided
- 1/4 cup fresh cilantro, chopped, divided (optional)
- 4 cups snow peas, trimmed and sliced on the bias
- 1 medium red bell pepper, thinly sliced
- 1/2 cup sesame seeds, toasted

Directions:

1. Place the spaghetti in a pot of boiling water and cook following the package directions until just softened, 8-10 minutes.
2. Transfer to a colander and rinse under in cold water. Drain.
3. In a large bowl, mix together the sesame oil, vinegar, canola oil, soy sauce, 1/4 cup scallions, crushed red pepper and 2 tablespoons cilantro (if using).

4. Add the bell peppers, snow peas and cooked noodles. Mix well to coat.

5. Sprinkle with sesame seeds and give a stir.

6. Place the spaghetti onto a serving plate, garnish with the chopped cilantro and remaining scallions.

7. Enjoy.

15. Beef and Vegetable Kebabs with Brown Rice

Prep time: 5 minutes

Cook time: 50 minutes

Nutritional information per serving: Calories 300; Fat 3 g; Cholesterol 39 mg.

Serves 2

Ingredients

- 1/2 cup brown rice
- 2 cups water
- 4 oz. (120 g) top sirloin
- 4 tablespoons fat-free Italian dressing
- 1 green pepper, seeded and cut into 4 pieces
- 4 cherry tomatoes
- 1 small onion, cut into 4 wedges
- 2 wooden skewers, soaked in water for 30 minutes, or metal skewers

Directions

1. Add the rice to a medium pot, pour in the water and bring to a boil over high heat.
2. Slow down the heat , put the lid on and simmer until the liquid is absorbed and the rice has softened, for 30-40 minutes. If needed, add more water to prevent the rice from sticking to the bottom.
3. Transfer the rice to a small bowl and keep covered to stay warm.
4. Cut the beef into 4 pieces and place in a small bowl. Sprinkle with Italian dressing refrigerate for at least 25 minutes to marinate, turning 2-3 times.

5. Preheat a gas grill or a broiler. Gently brush the grill rack or broiler pan with oil and set the rack 4-6 inches from the heat source.

6. Place 2 green pepper pieces, 2 cubes of meat, 2 onion wedges and 2 cherry tomatoes onto each skewer and transfer to the grill rack or broiler pan. Broil or grill the kebabs for 5 -10 minutes, turning 3-4 times.

7. Place the rice onto serving plates, put a 1 kebab on the top and serve immediately.

16. Red Lentil Curry

Prep time: 10 minutes

Cook time: 30 minutes

Nutritional information per serving: Calories 192; Fat 2.6 g; Cholesterol 0 mg.

Serves 8.

Ingredients:

- 2 cups red lentils
- 1 large onion, diced
- 1 tbs vegetable oil
- 2 tbs curry paste
- 1 tablespoon curry powder
- 1 tsp ground turmeric
- 1 tsp ground cumin
- 1 tsp chili powder
- 1 tsp salt
- 1 tsp white sugar
- 1 tsp minced garlic
- 1 tsp minced fresh ginger
- 1 (14.25 oz.) can tomato puree

Directions

1. Rinse the lentils under cold water and add to a large saucepan. Pour in enough water to cover and set over high heat.

2. Once it begins to boil, slow down the heat and let simmer, covered, until they are soft, about 18-20 minutes. You may

need to add more water during cooking to prevent lentils from sticking to the bottom. Drain.

3. Add the vegetable oil to a large frying pan and set over medium heat;add the onions and sauté, stirring frequently, until caramelized, for 15-18 minutes.

4. In a small bowl, mix together the curry paste, turmeric, chili powder, ginger curry powder, cumin, garlic, salt, and sugar, and add to the onions. Increase the heat stir-fry for 2 minutes, until fragrant.

5. Add the tomato puree and mix well. Pour the mixture over the lentils and stir well to coat.

Chapter 6 - Snack Recipes

1. Cinnamon French toast

Prep time: 3 minutes

Cook time: 10 minutes

Nutritional information per serving: Calories 295; Fat 2 g; Cholesterol 1 mg.

Serves 2

Ingredients

- 4 egg whites
- 1 teaspoon vanilla
- 1/8 teaspoon ground nutmeg
- 4 slices cinnamon bread
- 1/4 teaspoon ground cinnamon
- 2 teaspoons powdered sugar
- 1/4 cup maple syrup

Directions

1. In a small mixing bowl, beat the egg whites with nutmeg and vanilla. Whisk to mix evenly. Evenly coat the bread slices with the egg mixture.

2. Heat a nonstick skillet over medium heat. Once it is very hot, place the bread slices in the skillet and season with cinnamon.

3. Toast the bread for 3-5 minutes per side, until dark golden.

4. Put 2 slices of toast on serving plates, sprinkle with powdered sugar and maple syrup and enjoy.

2. Cauliflower Popcorn - Roasted Cauliflower

Prep time: 10 minutes

Cook time: 1 hr

Nutritional information per serving: Calories 156; Fat 12 g; Cholesterol 0 mg.

Serves 4.

Ingredients:

- 1 head cauliflower
- 4 tablespoons olive oil
- 1 teaspoon salt, to taste

Directions:

1. Preheat oven to 425 F (220 C).

2. Core the cauliflower and remove thick stems. Chop the florets into not very small pieces.

3. Add the olive oil and salt to a large bowl and stir well. Add the chopped cauliflower to the oil mixture and toss well to coat.

4. Lightly coat the baking dish with oil or line with parchment. Arrange the cauliflower pieces on the prepared baking sheet and roast in the oven for 50-60 minutes, turning occasionally, until most of them acquire golden crust. Serve hot and enjoy.

3. Parmesan Potato Pancakes

Prep time: 10 minutes

Cook time: 12 minutes

Nutritional information per serving: Calories 150; Fat 4 g; Cholesterol 4 mg.

Serves 4.

Ingredients:

- 2 cups leftover mashed potatoes
- 2 tablespoons chopped fresh chives or green onions
- 1 large egg white
- 1/4 cup seasoned breadcrumbs, divided
- 2 tablespoons grated fresh Parmesan cheese
- 2 teaspoons olive oil, divided

Directions:

1. In a medium bowl, mix together the egg white, potatoes, 2 tablespoons breadcrumbs and chives.

2. Place the cheese and 2 tablespoons breadcrumbs in a small plate and mix with fingers. Shape 8 medium patties, coat with breadcrumb mixture and place in a platter.

3. Add 1 teaspoon oil to a large frying pan and set over medium-high heat. Fry the patties in 2 batches, 4 at a time. Add the patties to the pan and cook for 4-5 minutes per side or until light brown. Great to serve patties with low fat sour cream.

4. Italian Bruschetta

Prep time: 12minutes

Cook time:3 minutes

Nutritional information per serving: Calories 119; Fat 4 g; Cholesterol 0 mg.

Serves 16

Ingredients:

- 1 French baguette
- 1/4 cup basil, chopped
- 6 Roma tomatoes, chopped
- 3 cloves garlic, chopped, plus 1 whole clove for rubbing)
- 1/4 cup olive oil
- 1/2 tsp salt

Directions:

1. Thinly slice the baguette and broil for 3-4 minutes until golden and crispy. Remove from the oven and let cool.

2. In a small bowl, place together the tomatoes, chopped garlic, basil and olive oil, season with salt.

3. Remove the ends of the whole garlic clove. Rub each slice of the toasted baguette with garlic. Spoon little amount of tomato mixture on the bread and spread evenly

4. Place the done slices on a flat platter and serve immediately..

5. Crispy Zucchini Sticks

Prep time: 12minutes

Cook time:3 minutes

Nutritional information per serving: Calories 49; Fat 2.9 g; Cholesterol 2 mg.

Serves 8

Ingredients

- 4 zucchini, medium
- 1 cup red bell pepper, minced
- 1/2 cup tomatoes, minced
- 1/2 cup Kalamata olives, pitted & minced
- 1/4 cup garlic, minced
- 4 tbsp oregano, dried
- 1 tsp black pepper
- 1/4 cup feta cheese, crumbled
- 1/4 cup parsley, finely chopped

Directions:

1. Preheat oven to 350 F (170 C). Halve the zucchini in lengthwise and using a spoon, scoop out the middle part. Set aside.

2. Place the olives, tomato, garlic, bell pepper, oregano and black pepper in a medium bowl and stir to combine.

3. Evenly spoon the mixture into holed zucchini. Arrange the zucchini on a baking dish and bake in the preheated oven. Sprinkle the stiffed zucchini with crumbled cheese, broil for 2-3 minutes on HIGH until the cheese is melted and lightly browned.

4. Withdraw from the oven, garnish with chopped parsley.

5. Can be served warm, hot or cold.

6. Fruity Fun Skewers

Prep time: 15 minutes

Cook time: 0 minute

Nutritional information per serving: Calories 61; Fat 0.3 g; Cholesterol 0 mg.

Serves 5.

- 5 large strawberries, halved
- 1/4 cantaloupe, cut into balls or cubes
- 2 bananas, peeled and cut into chunks
- 1 apple, cut into chunks
- 20 skewers

Directions

1. Alternately thread the cantaloupe, apple pieces, strawberries, banana onto the skewers. Make sure to put at least 2 pieces of fruit on each skewer.
2. Place the fruit skewers on a serving platter and enjoy.

7. Baked Sweet Potato Sticks

Prep time: 15 minutes

Cook time: 40 minutes

Nutritional information per serving: Calories 132; Fat 1.9 g; Cholesterol 0 mg.

Serves 8.

Ingredients:

- 1 tablespoon olive oil
- 1/2 teaspoon paprika
- 8 sweet potatoes, sliced lengthwise into quarters

Directions:

1. Preheat oven to 400 F (200 C). Gently coat a baking sheet with olive oil.

2. Combine the olive oil and paprika in a large bowl, add the sliced potato, and mix with hands to coat evenly. Transfer to the prepared baking sheet and place in the preheated oven.

3. Bake for 40 minutes or until the potatoes acquire golden crust.

8. Corn and Garbanzo Bean Patties

Prep time: 5 minutes

Cook time: 10 minutes

Nutritional information per serving: Calories 370; Fat 2.3 g; Cholesterol 0 mg.

Serves 6

Ingredients:

- 1 tbs canola oil
- 1 1/2 cups fresh or frozen corn kernels (thawed)
- 2 tbs shallots, chopped
- 1/2 tsp oregano, ground
- 2 tsp fresh Italian parsley, minced
- 1 (19 oz./230 g) can garbanzo beans, drained
- 1 cup fresh French breadcrumbs
- 2 tbs fine grain cornmeal or 2 tablespoons masa harina
- 1/2 teaspoon salt
- 2 tbs red bell peppers, minced
- 1 tbs polenta (coarse cornmeal)

Dressing

- 1/4 cup fresh lemon juice
- 1/3 cup extra virgin olive oil
- Salt (to taste)
- Fresh ground black pepper, to taste
- Garnish
- 5 oz. (150 g) arugula leaves
- Fresh garlic chives, minced

Directions:

1. Add 1 teaspoon of olive oil to a large skillet and set over medium-high heat. Stir in the shallots, corn, and oregano and cook for a couple of minutes. Remove from the heat and let cool. Then add the fresh parsley and stir to combine.

2. Place the cornmeal, garbanzo beans, 2 tablespoons of the reserved garbanzo bean liquid, French bread crumbs, minced red bell pepper and salt in a blender. Process until coarsely ground. Then add the fried corn and shallot mixture, another tablespoon of bean liquid and process, about 8-10 times until finely ground.

3. Moisten your hands and shape 6 patties. Gently coat the patties with polenta and fry in the remaining 1 tablespoon of olive oil over medium to high heat. Cook the patties in batches, 3 at a time. Let them cook for 5 minutes per side until brown on all sides.

4. Place the cooked patties in the oven at 200 °F (100 °C) to keep warm.

5. Make the dressing by combining fresh lemon juice, the olive oil, salt and pepper in a small cup.

6. Drizzle the mixture over the arugula and slightly toss to coat. Divide the herbs among six serving bowls and top with cooked patties. Decorate with fresh chives, and serve immediately with the remaining dressing.

9. Turkey & Tomato Panini

Prep time: 5 minutes

Cook time: 5 minutes

Nutritional information per serving: Calories 286; Fat 6 g; Cholesterol 27 mg.

Serves 4.

Ingredients:

- 3 tbs reduced-fat mayonnaise
- 2 tbs nonfat plain yogurt
- 2 tbs Parmesan cheese, shredded
- 2 tbs chopped fresh basil
- 1 tsp lemon juice
- Freshly ground pepper, to taste
- 8 slices whole-wheat bread
- 8 oz. (230 g) reduced-sodium deli turkey, thinly sliced
- 8 tomato slices
- 2 tsp canola oil

Directions:

1. In a small bowl, mix together the Parmesan, mayonnaise, lemon juice, yogurt, basil, and pepper.

2. Coat one side of each slice of bread with 2 teaspoons of the mixture on each slice of bread. Top 4 slices of bread with turkey and tomato slices and cover with the remaining bread, coated side down.

3. Add 1 teaspoon oil to a large frying pan and set over medium heat. Place 2 panini in the pan, press with spoons and cook for 2 minutes, until golden.

4.   Flip to brown the other side. Once theses two paninis are done, add the remaining 1 teaspoon oil to the pan and cook the next 2.

10. Roasted Asparagus

Prep Time: 10 minutes

Cook Time: 15 minutes

Nutritional information per serving: Calories 68, Fat 5 g, Cholesterol 0 mg.

Serves 4.

Ingredients:

- 1 lb asparagus
- 1 1/2 tablespoons olive oil
- 1/2 teaspoon kosher salt (or 1/4 teaspoon regular table salt)

Directions:

1. Preheat oven to 425°F (220 °C).
2. Remove the woody root ends of the asparagus spears. Slightly peel off the bottom part of the spears and rinse in the cold water. Drain the asparagus and place on a baking sheet lined with foil.
3. Season with salt and drizzle with olive oil.
4. Roast in the oven for 10-12 minutes or to your desired doneness. Great served with a light vinaigrette.

11. Sautéed Broccoli

Prep Time: 10 minutes

Cook Time: 7 minutes

Nutritional information per serving: Calories 108.5, Fat 8 g, Cholesterol 0 mg.

Serves 4.

Ingredients:

- 3 tablespoons water
- 1/4 teaspoon salt
- 1/8 teaspoon pepper (I used garlic pepper blend)
- 2 tablespoons vegetable oil
- 1 1/4 lbs broccoli, separated into small florets and stems, sliced

Directions:

1. In a small cup, mix together the salt, pepper and water.

2. Heat the oil in a large frying pan over medium-high heat. Add the broccoli stems and fry for 2 minutes, without stirring, until lightly golden. Add the florets, give a stir and fry for another 2-3 minutes, again without stirring.

3. Pour the spicy water over the broccoli and cook for 3 minutes, covered. Add water spice mixture and cover pan with lid, cooking for two minutes. Remove the lid, cook for another 1-2 minutes and remove from the heat.

12. Marinated Feta and Olive Skewers

Prep Time: **25** minutes
Nutritional information per serving: Calories 59,Fat 5 g,Cholesterol 0 mg.

Serves 8

Ingredients:

- 2 tsp fennel seeds
- 2 tsp orange zest
- 3 tbs fresh orange juice
- 1 tsp freshly ground black pepper
- 4 oz. (120 g) feta cheese, cut into 24 (1/2-inch) cubes
- 24 (6-inch) wooden skewers
- 24 fresh mint leaves
- 12 pitted green olives, halved
- 1/4 large English cucumber, seeded and cut

Directions:

1. In a medium bowl, mix together the orange zest and juice, fennel seeds, and pepper.

2. Add the cut feta and marinate for about an hour at room temperature or up to 4 hours in the refrigerator.

3. Alternately thread 1 mint leaf, 1 cucumber chunk and 1 olive half on a skewer. Put 1 piece of feta on the end.

4. You can thread skewers in advance and store them in the refrigerator until serving. Remove from the fridge 10-15 minutes before the serving.

13. Arugula and Goat Cheese Pizza

Prep Time: 10 minutes
Cook Time:18 minutes
Nutritional information per serving: Calories 295,Fat 10 g,Cholesterol 5 mg.

Serves 4

Ingredients:

- 1/4 cup walnuts, coarsely chopped
- 2 tsp olive oil, divided
- 1 cup thinly sliced red onion
- 1 (8-oz. /320 g) whole-wheat pizza crust
- 1 cup grape tomatoes, halved
- 1/4 tsp salt
- 1/4 tsp freshly ground black pepper
- 1 1/2 oz. (40 g) goat cheese, sliced
- 3/4 cup loosely packed baby arugula

Directions:

1. Preheat oven to 450°F (220 °C).

2. Place the walnuts on a baking sheet and toast for about 5 minutes or until lightly brown and fragrant. Remove from the pan and let cool.

3. Add 1 teaspoon oil to a frying pan and set over medium heat. Add the onion and sauté, stirring occasionally, 7 minutes or until onion is golden and tender.

4. Put the crust on a baking sheet brushed with cooking spray.

5. Place the tomatoes, onion and walnuts. Sprinkle with salt and pepper and put goat cheese slices on the top.

6. Bake in the oven for 6-7 minutes, until the edges of crust are golden and crispy, Drizzle the pizza with the remaining oil

and top with arugula. Let stand for 10 minutes, then cut into wedges and serve.

14. Grilled Zucchini Roll-Ups with Herbs and Cheese

Prep Time: 10 minutes
Cook Time:10 minutes
Nutritional information per serving: Calories 80,Fat 6 g,Cholesterol 5 mg.

Serves 4

Ingredients:

- 1 tbs olive oil
- 1/8 tsp salt, plus more to taste
- 1/16 tsp of freshly ground black pepper, plus more to taste
- 1 1/2 oz. (40 g) fresh goat cheese
- 1 tbs fresh parsley, chopped
- 1/2 tsp fresh lemon juice
- 3 small zucchini (about 1/2 pound each), thinly sliced lengthwise
- 2 oz. (60 g) bagged baby spinach
- 1/3 cup basil leaves

Directions:

1. Preheat grill or grill pan to medium.
2. Coat the zucchini slices with oil on both sides and season with salt and pepper. Grill 3-4 minutes per side until soft and golden.
3. Place the parsley, goat cheese, and lemon juice in a small bowl, mix together, crumbling with a fork.
4. Place about 1/2 teaspoon of the cheese mixture about at the end of a zucchini slice. Add a few spinach leaves and a small basil leaf on the top.

5. Fold the slice and place on a serving plate seam side down. In this way fold the remaining zucchini slices.

6. Zucchini roll-ups can be made a day before and kept in the refrigerator.

15. Vanilla-Lemon Berry Parfaits

Prep Time: 10 minutes
Nutritional information per serving: Calories 176,Fat 2 g,Cholesterol 10 mg.

Serves 4

Ingredients:

- 1 cup plain low-fat yogurt
- 2 (3.5-ounce) containers fat-free vanilla pudding
- 2 tbs bottled lemon curd
- 1/2 tsp vanilla extract
- 2 tbs honey
- Zest of 1 lemon
- 1 tbs fresh lemon juice
- 3 cups mixed berries (such as blueberries, strawberries, and raspberries)
- Fresh mint leaves (optional)

Directions:

1. Place the pudding, yogurt, vanilla extract and lemon curd in a small bowl, mix to combine and set aside.
2. In a separate bowl, combine the lemon zest, lemon and juice honey. Toss in the mixed berries and gently mix to coat.
3. Add 3 tablespoons of the yogurt mixture into each serving glass, add 1/4 cup of the berries, then add another 3 tablespoons yogurt on the top, and another 1/4 cup berries.
4. Garnish the mixture with fresh mint and serve immediately.

Conclusion

Thank you again for buying this book!

I hope this book was helpful and valuable in changing your spirit and approach to your own health. Again, you should remember; whatever you want to change, you should start changing yourself. It's half the battle towards success.

The guidance and recipes provided in this book hopefully has helped you in achieving your goal in reducing the cholesterol and bringing back full health to your body. I believe that the success of your work will bring impact on your entire life, making you more positive and active which again are the main guarantees regarding health. This book doesn't target any specific social group (youth, men, women, etc) and includes information that can be used and absorbed by anyone who is not indifferent towards his/her health.

And finally, the book was designed in the most accessible manner and form to make your time in kitchen and life not only healthier but also pleasant.

Finally, if you enjoyed this book, please take the time to share your thoughts and post a review on Amazon. It'd be greatly appreciated!

Thank you and good luck in your future achievements!

Printed in Great Britain
by Amazon.co.uk, Ltd.,
Marston Gate.